Cat Scratch Disease

Causes, Transmission, Symptoms, Diagnosis and Treatment of Cat Scratch Disease

By:

Chris Williams

Table of Contents

Chapter. 1

Introduction

1.1 Definition of Cat Scratch Disease (CSD)

Cat Scratch Disease (CSD) is a bacterial infection primarily caused by the bacterium *Bartonella henselae*. This disease typically manifests following a scratch or bite from an infected cat. While cats are the primary reservoirs for the bacteria, transmission to humans occurs through contact with the cat's saliva via scratches or bites, or through exposure to their fur. The disease usually presents itself with mild symptoms, including a bump or blister at the site of injury, along with swollen lymph nodes, fever, fatigue, headache, and general malaise.

1.2 Overview of its significance

Cat Scratch Disease (CSD) holds significance due to its prevalence, though it is often a relatively mild illness. Its importance lies in several aspects:

- Common Occurrence: CSD is a relatively common infection, especially among children and pet owners who have close contact with cats. The CDC estimates thousands of new cases in the United States annually.
- Health Impact: While typically mild and self-limiting, CSD can cause discomfort with symptoms such as swollen lymph nodes, fever, and malaise. In rare cases, it can lead to severe complications, especially in immunocompromised individuals.
- Risk Groups: Children and individuals with weakened immune systems are at higher risk of experiencing more severe symptoms or complications if infected.

- Diagnostic Challenges: Diagnosing CSD can sometimes be challenging due to the non-specific nature of its symptoms and the need for specialized tests to confirm the presence of the bacteria.
- Public Health Awareness: Educating the public, especially pet owners and healthcare providers, about the risks, symptoms, and preventive measures is crucial to prevent and manage CSD cases effectively.
- One Health Perspective: As a zoonotic disease, CSD highlights the interconnectedness of human and animal health, emphasizing the importance of responsible pet ownership and veterinary care to minimize the risk of transmission.

Chapter. 2

Causes of Cat Scratch Disease

2.1 Bacterial origin *(Bartonella henselae)*

Bartonella henselae serves as the primary causative agent behind Cat Scratch Disease (CSD). This bacterium is transmitted primarily through the scratch or bite of an infected cat, especially kittens. Once inside the human body, *Bartonella henselae* leads to the development of CSD. When an infected cat scratches or bites a person, the bacterium present in the cat's saliva or on its claws enters the human body. Once inside, it causes an immune response that leads to the characteristic symptoms of CSD, such as swollen lymph nodes, fever, headache, and fatigue. Although cats are the primary reservoir for *Bartonella henselae,* transmission to humans can also occur through flea bites or by accidental ingestion of flea feces containing the bacterium.

2.2 Transmission from cats to humans

Transmission of Cat Scratch Disease (CSD) from cats to humans primarily occurs through direct contact with an infected cat's saliva through a scratch or bite. The process involves the following steps:

- Scratches or Bites: Cats infected with *Bartonella henselae* may not display symptoms but can carry the bacteria. When an infected cat scratches or bites a person, the bacteria in its saliva or on its claws can enter the human body.
- Skin Breakage: The bacteria present on the cat's claws or teeth can penetrate the skin during a scratch or bite, leading to the introduction of *Bartonella henselae* into the human system.
- Contact with Cat's Saliva: Even without visible scratches, contact with a cat's saliva, particularly when it comes into contact with broken skin or mucous membranes

(like the eyes or mouth), can transmit the bacteria.

- Flea Vector: In some cases, transmission might also occur indirectly through flea bites or contact with flea feces carrying the bacteria. Cats can be infected with *Bartonella henselae* through fleas, and when a person is bitten by an infected flea or inadvertently ingests flea dirt, transmission can occur.

2.3 Risk factors for contracting CSD

Several risk factors increase the likelihood of contracting Cat Scratch Disease (CSD). These include:

- Cat Exposure: Close contact with cats, especially kittens, that might carry *Bartonella henselae* bacteria increases the risk. Cats that spend time outdoors or in multi-cat environments have a higher likelihood of carrying the bacterium.

- Cat Scratch or Bite: Direct contact with a scratch or bite from an infected cat is a significant risk factor for contracting CSD.

- Immune System Status: Individuals with compromised immune systems, such as those with HIV/AIDS, undergoing chemotherapy, or taking immunosuppressant medications, are at higher risk of developing severe forms of CSD if infected.

- Age: Children, particularly those under the age of 15, are more likely to contract CSD due to their propensity for interacting closely with pets and potentially being less aware of safety precautions around cats.

- Not practicing good hygiene: Failure to wash hands properly after handling cats, especially before touching the face or

consuming food, increases the risk
of contracting CSD.

Chapter. 3

Symptoms of Cat Scratch Disease

3.1 Early symptoms after exposure

Following exposure to *Bartonella henselae*, the bacterium responsible for Cat Scratch Disease (CSD), early symptoms may begin to manifest within 3-14 days, though this timeframe can vary. The initial symptoms can include:

- Redness and Swelling: The area where the scratch or bite occurred might develop redness, tenderness, and swelling. A small bump or blister may form at the site of injury.
- Lymph Node Swelling: Swelling of nearby lymph nodes, particularly those closest to the site of the scratch or bite, is a common early symptom. This swelling can persist for several weeks.

- Mild Fever: Some individuals may experience a mild fever, along with other non-specific flu-like symptoms such as fatigue, headache, and general malaise.

3.2 Progression of symptoms

The initial exposure to *Bartonella henselae*, the progression of Cat Scratch Disease (CSD) symptoms can vary in individuals. The symptoms typically evolve over several weeks and might include:

- Continued Swelling: The lymph nodes near the site of the scratch or bite may continue to enlarge and become more painful, this swelling might persist for several weeks.
- Fever and Fatigue: Mild fever, along with ongoing fatigue, might persist or fluctuate throughout the course of the illness.
- Flu-like Symptoms: Some individuals might experience flu-

like symptoms such as headache, malaise, and overall discomfort.

- Appearance of Lesions: In a small percentage of cases, additional symptoms like skin lesions, especially erythematous nodules or papules, might develop at the site of the scratch or bite or in other areas of the body.
- Rare Complications: In rare instances, more severe complications can occur, especially in immunocompromised individuals, which might involve prolonged fever, severe headaches, joint pain, and, in very rare cases, involvement of internal organs.

3.3 Severity and variations in symptoms

Cat Scratch Disease (CSD) symptoms can vary widely in severity and presentation among individuals. Some experience a mild form of the disease, while others might have more severe manifestations. Variations in symptoms include:

- Mild Cases: Many individuals have mild symptoms resembling a mild infection or flu-like illness. These can include a small bump or blister at the site of the scratch or bite, along with swollen and tender lymph nodes. Fever, fatigue, headache, and malaise may also be present but are typically mild and self-limiting.
- Moderate Cases: Some people might experience more pronounced symptoms, including larger and more painful lymph node swelling, prolonged fever, and more intense flu-like symptoms. Skin lesions might develop at the site of the injury.
- Severe Cases: Although uncommon, in rare instances, Cat Scratch Disease can lead to severe complications, particularly in immunocompromised individuals. This might involve persistent high fever, severe headaches, joint pain,

and even involvement of internal organs. Such cases might require specialized medical attention and treatment.

- Asymptomatic Cases: In some instances, individuals exposed to Bartonella henselae might not exhibit any noticeable symptoms at all.

Chapter. 4

Diagnosis of Cat Scratch Disease

4.1 Clinical examination

Clinical examination for Cat Scratch Disease (CSD) typically involves several steps:

- Medical History: The healthcare provider will inquire about recent interactions with cats, especially any scratches or bites, and the onset of symptoms.
- Physical Examination: A physical examination will focus on assessing lymph nodes for enlargement, tenderness, and warmth, particularly in areas near the scratch or bite. The site of the injury might also be examined for signs of inflammation or infection.

- Laboratory Tests: In some cases, additional tests might be ordered to support the diagnosis, such as:

☐ Blood tests: To check for an increase in specific antibodies against Bartonella henselae.

☐ Biopsy of lymph nodes: Rarely, if necessary, a sample of an enlarged lymph node might be taken for examination to confirm the presence of the bacteria.

- Imaging Studies: Imaging tests like ultrasound or CT scans might be recommended in severe or complicated cases to assess the extent of lymph node involvement or if internal organ complications are suspected.

- Differential Diagnosis: The healthcare provider might also consider other conditions with similar symptoms, such as bacterial or viral infections, lymphadenitis, or other causes of lymph node enlargement.

4.2 Laboratory tests for confirmation

Laboratory tests play a crucial role in confirming Cat Scratch Disease (CSD) diagnosis. Some of the key laboratory tests used for confirmation include:

- Serological Tests: These tests detect antibodies produced by the body in response to *Bartonella henselae* infection. Enzyme-linked immunosorbent assay (ELISA) and indirect fluorescent antibody (IFA) tests are commonly used to detect these antibodies in blood samples.
- PCR (Polymerase Chain Reaction): PCR tests are used to detect the genetic material (DNA) of *Bartonella henselae* in blood, tissue samples, or lymph node aspirates. This test can provide a more direct confirmation of the presence of the bacterium.
- Culture Tests: Culturing *Bartonella henselae* from clinical samples (such as lymph node

aspirates or biopsies) is possible but challenging and often not routinely performed due to the difficulty in culturing the bacteria.

- Histopathology: Examination of lymph node biopsy samples under a microscope can reveal characteristic changes, such as granulomatous inflammation, which support the diagnosis of CSD.

4.3 Differential diagnoses

Several conditions can present with symptoms similar to Cat Scratch Disease (CSD). Differential diagnoses include:

- Bacterial Infections: Other bacterial infections, such as staphylococcal or streptococcal infections, can cause lymph node enlargement and skin manifestations resembling CSD.
- Viral Infections: Viral illnesses like infectious mononucleosis

(caused by Epstein-Barr virus) and adenovirus infections can also lead to swollen lymph nodes and flu-like symptoms.

- Tuberculosis: Tuberculous lymphadenitis can present with enlarged lymph nodes and sometimes skin lesions, mimicking CSD.
- Fungal Infections: Certain fungal infections, such as sporotrichosis, can cause skin lesions and lymph node swelling similar to CSD.
- Lymphoma: Lymphoma, a type of cancer affecting the lymphatic system, can manifest with enlarged lymph nodes and constitutional symptoms, which might resemble CSD.
- Toxoplasmosis: This parasitic infection can cause lymph node enlargement and flu-like symptoms, potentially resembling CSD.

Chapter. 5

Treatment of Cat Scratch Disease

5.1 Symptomatic management

Symptomatic management of Cat Scratch Disease (CSD) focuses on alleviating discomfort and addressing specific symptoms. Here are some approaches to manage symptoms associated with CSD:

- Pain and Inflammation: Over-the-counter pain relievers such as acetaminophen (Tylenol) or nonsteroidal anti-inflammatory drugs (NSAIDs) like ibuprofen (Advil, Motrin) may help reduce pain and inflammation associated with swollen lymph nodes.
- Fever: Fever-reducing medications like acetaminophen or ibuprofen can also help manage fever if it's causing discomfort.

- Localized Care: Proper wound care of the scratch or bite site is essential to prevent infection. Cleaning the area with soap and water, applying antibiotic ointment, and covering it with a bandage can aid in healing and prevent secondary infections.
- Rest and Hydration: Adequate rest and staying hydrated by drinking plenty of fluids can support the body's immune response and recovery.
- Observation: Regular monitoring of symptoms and seeking medical attention if symptoms worsen or persist is crucial, especially in severe or prolonged cases of CSD or in individuals with weakened immune systems.

5.2 Antibiotic treatment

Antibiotic treatment is generally recommended for severe cases of CSD, immunocompromised individuals, or when there's involvement of other organs or complications. It's essential to complete the full course of antibiotics as prescribed by the healthcare provider to ensure the complete eradication of the infection.

- Azithromycin: This is often considered the first-line antibiotic for CSD. A typical course may last from 5 to 14 days, depending on the severity of symptoms.
- Doxycycline: It might be used as an alternative treatment, especially in cases where azithromycin cannot be administered. Treatment duration may vary based on the healthcare provider's recommendation.
- Trimethoprim-sulfamethoxazole (TMP-SMX): This antibiotic combination might be prescribed for CSD treatment, especially in individuals who cannot tolerate other antibiotics.

5.3 Complications and management strategies

Cat Scratch Disease resolves on its own without complications in most cases. However, in rare instances or in individuals with weakened immune systems, complications can arise.

Potential complications include:

- Parinaud's Oculoglandular Syndrome: This complication involves inflammation of the conjunctiva of the eye and nearby lymph nodes. It might cause redness, irritation, and swelling around the eye.
- Neurological Complications: In extremely rare cases, CSD can lead to neurological complications such as encephalitis, seizures, or other neurological issues.
- Systemic Involvement: Severe or disseminated infections can affect various organs or systems in the body, leading to a more complex disease course.

Management strategies for complications of CSD involve:

- Medical Evaluation: Immediate medical evaluation is crucial if complications are suspected or symptoms worsen, especially in immunocompromised individuals or if neurological symptoms develop.
- Specialized Treatment: Complicated cases might require specialized medical care, including specific treatments targeted at managing the complications. Neurological complications, for instance, might require interventions by neurologists or infectious disease specialists.
- Supportive Care: Supportive care to manage symptoms and complications might involve medications to alleviate pain,

inflammation, or other specific symptoms.

- Follow-up Care: Close monitoring and follow-up with healthcare providers are essential to ensure proper management and resolution of complications.

Chapter. 6

Prevention of Cat Scratch Disease

6.1 Hygiene practices after cat interaction

Practicing good hygiene after interacting with cats is essential to minimize the risk of contracting Cat Scratch Disease (CSD) and other potential infections. Some hygiene practices to follow are listed below:

- Handwashing: Wash hands thoroughly with soap and water after handling cats, especially before touching your face, eating, or preparing food. Handwashing for at least 20 seconds helps eliminate bacteria and reduces the risk of infection.
- Avoid Face Contact: Avoid touching your face, especially your eyes, nose, and mouth, after handling cats, as this can

potentially transfer bacteria from the cat's fur or saliva.

- Wound Care: Immediately clean any scratches or bites from cats with soap and water. Apply an antiseptic and cover the wound with a clean bandage to prevent infection.
- Avoid Aggravating Cats: Be mindful of cats' behaviors and avoid actions that could potentially cause scratches or bites, especially from kittens who might playfully scratch or bite.
- Flea Control: Regularly use flea control products recommended by veterinarians to minimize the risk of fleas transmitting *Bartonella henselae* between cats and humans.
- Regular Veterinary Care: Ensure cats receive routine veterinary care, including vaccinations and regular check-ups, to maintain their health and reduce the

likelihood of transmitting infections.

- Educational Measures: Teach children proper handling of cats to minimize the risk of scratches or bites. Encourage hand washing after interacting with pets.

6.2 Controlling exposure to fleas on cats

Fleas controlling on cats is essential not only for their health but also to reduce the risk of transmitting *Bartonella henselae,* The effective strategies to control fleas on cats are listed below:

- Regular Veterinary Care: Schedule routine check-ups with a veterinarian. They can recommend appropriate flea control products, such as topical treatments, oral medications, or flea collars, based on your cat's age, health status, and environment.
- Use Flea Preventatives: Administer flea control products

recommended by your veterinarian consistently and as directed. These products can prevent fleas from infesting your cat and home.

- Environmental Management: Regularly vacuum areas where your cat spends time, such as carpets, furniture, and bedding. Wash pet bedding in hot water to kill flea eggs, larvae, and adults.
- Outdoor Control: Minimize outdoor exposure if possible, especially in areas known for high flea populations. Consider limiting your cat's outdoor access or using preventive measures if they spend time outdoors.
- Household Treatment: Use flea control products specifically designed for homes, like sprays or foggers, to target flea eggs and larvae in your living space.
- Consult a Professional: If your home experiences a severe flea infestation, seek advice from pest

control professionals for effective and safe treatment options.

6.3 Educating about risks and precautions

Educating individuals, especially pet owners and those in close contact with cats, about the risks and precautions associated with Cat Scratch Disease (CSD) is crucial in preventing its transmission:

- Understanding Transmission: Explain how CSD is transmitted, primarily through scratches or bites from infected cats, and sometimes through fleas carrying the bacteria.
- High-Risk Activities: Highlight activities that might increase the risk of contracting CSD, such as rough play with cats, particularly kittens, and inadequate hand hygiene after handling cats.
- Hygiene Practices: Emphasize the importance of handwashing with soap and water after handling cats,

especially before eating or touching the face. Encourage cleaning and covering any cat scratches or bites promptly.

- Flea Control: Stress the significance of regular flea control measures for cats to reduce the risk of *Bartonella henselae* transmission through flea bites.
- Monitoring and Seeking Medical Attention: Educate about monitoring any scratches or bites for signs of infection and seeking medical advice if symptoms develop or worsen.
- Awareness in Vulnerable Groups: Highlight the increased risk of severe CSD in children and individuals with weakened immune systems, stressing the importance of extra precautions and prompt medical attention for them.
- Veterinary Care: Encourage regular veterinary care for cats,

including vaccinations, flea control, and routine check-ups.

- First Aid for Wounds: Educate about proper first aid for cat scratches or bites, including cleaning the wound thoroughly with soap and water and applying antiseptic.
- Responsible Pet Ownership: Encourage responsible pet ownership, including vaccinations, regular check-ups, and minimizing rough play that might lead to scratches or bites.
- Awareness Campaigns: Utilize posters, brochures, online resources, and community events to raise awareness about CSD and preventive measures.

Conclusion

Most cases of CSD resolve without treatment within a few weeks to a few months. However, in some instances, complications can occur, such as prolonged fever, abscess formation, or involvement of other organs. Seeking medical attention is advisable if symptoms persist or worsen.